# COMPLETE INTERMITTENT FASTING BOOK

## The Complete guide to a 30 Day Intermittent Fasting

Kaya K. Welch

*"Nature is the physician of man"*

*This quote by Hippocrates, known as the father of modern medicine, speaks to the idea that the natural world holds many of the answers to our health and wellness. Intermittent fasting is a natural and ancient practice that has been used by humans for centuries, and it has the potential to improve our health and wellbeing in many ways. By tapping into the power of our own bodies and working with the natural rhythms of our physiology, we can unlock a range of benefits that support our overall health and wellness.*

HIPPOCRATES

# CONTENTS

# PREFACE

Welcome to the complete intermittent fasting book! I have seen the transformative effects that intermittent fasting can have on people's health and wellness. But before we dive into the specifics of how to do intermittent fasting, I want to take a moment to reflect on the bigger picture.

The truth is, there is no one-size-fits-all approach to health and wellness. What works for one person may not work for another, and what is healthy for one person may not be healthy for another. This is why it is so important to approach intermittent fasting with an open mind and a willingness to experiment and learn.

In this book, we will explore the science behind intermittent fasting, the different types of fasting, and the potential benefits and risks associated with this approach. We will also provide practical tips and tools for getting started with intermittent fasting, including meal plans, recipes, and strategies for dealing with hunger and cravings.

But more than anything, this book is about helping you to develop a healthy and sustainable relationship with food and your body. By learning to listen to your body's signals and needs, you can create a lifestyle that supports your overall health and wellness goals.

So whether you are looking to lose weight, improve your metabolic health, or simply feel better in your own skin, I hope that this book will provide you with the information and inspiration you need to start your own intermittent fasting journey. Remember, this is a marathon, not a sprint, and the key to success is consistency, patience, and self-compassion. Let's get started!

# INTRODUCTION

Intermittent fasting is a dietary approach that has gained popularity in recent years for its potential benefits in weight loss, improved health markers, and longevity. The practice of intermittent fasting involves cycling between periods of eating and fasting, with the goal of consuming food within a specific time window each day. The duration and frequency of fasting can vary widely depending on the chosen method of intermittent fasting.

In this guide, we will explore a 30-day approach to intermittent fasting and how it can benefit your health. We will cover the science behind intermittent fasting and the different types of fasting methods to help you choose the right approach for your goals and lifestyle. We will also discuss the potential risks and side effects of intermittent fasting and how to prepare yourself mentally and physically for the challenge.

Getting started with intermittent fasting can be overwhelming, but we will provide practical tips and strategies to help you navigate your fasting journey. We will guide you through creating a fasting schedule that fits your lifestyle, setting realistic goals, and handling cravings and hunger during your fasting window.

Eating a healthy and balanced diet during your eating window is essential to optimize the benefits of intermittent fasting. In chapter three, we will provide you with recipes and meal ideas to ensure that you are getting the nutrients you need to support your health and weight loss goals.

We will also discuss how to make intermittent fasting a sustainable lifestyle choice beyond the 30-day period, including strategies for maintaining a healthy diet and lifestyle outside of your fasting window and incorporating exercise to support your overall health.

Lastly, we will address common challenges and roadblocks that may arise during your fasting journey, and provide troubleshooting strategies to help you overcome them.

By the end of this guide, you will have a thorough understanding of intermittent fasting and how to incorporate it into your life for optimal health and wellness. So, let's get started on your 30-day intermittent fasting journey.

# UNDERSTANDING INTERMITTENT FASTING

*The Science, Types and Side effects*

## *The science behind intermittent fasting and its benefits*

Intermittent fasting (IF) is a dietary pattern that involves alternating periods of fasting and feeding. It has become increasingly popular in recent years due to its potential health benefits beyond just weight loss. In this chapter, we will delve into the science behind IF and the benefits it can provide for your overall health.

One of the main physiological changes that occur during IF is the depletion of glycogen stores in the liver and muscles. This triggers the body to shift from using glucose as its primary fuel source to using stored fats for energy. As a result, the body enters a state of ketosis, where it produces ketone bodies that can provide energy to the brain and other organs.

IF has been shown to improve insulin sensitivity, which is the ability of your body to respond to insulin and regulate blood sugar levels. This can be beneficial for people with type 2 diabetes or prediabetes, as it can improve their blood sugar control and reduce their risk of developing diabetes-related complications.

IF has also been shown to reduce inflammation in the body, which is a common factor in many chronic diseases. It does this by decreasing the production of pro-inflammatory cytokines and increasing the production of anti-inflammatory cytokines.

Studies have shown that IF can have positive effects on heart health by reducing blood pressure, total cholesterol, and LDL (bad) cholesterol levels. It may also improve triglyceride levels, which are another important risk factor for heart disease.

In addition to the physical benefits, IF has been shown to

have positive effects on cognitive function and brain health. Studies have demonstrated improvements in memory, focus, and concentration, as well as a reduction in the risk of neurodegenerative diseases such as Alzheimer's and Parkinson's.

Finally, IF may offer protection against cancer by reducing oxidative stress, inflammation, and insulin levels, all of which are factors that can contribute to the development of cancer.

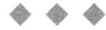

Overall, the science behind IF suggests that it can offer numerous health benefits beyond just weight loss. However, it's important to note that more research is needed to fully understand the effects of IF on different populations and in the long term.

# *The different types of intermittent fasting and how to choose the right one for you*

Intermittent fasting is not a one-size-fits-all approach, and there are different types of intermittent fasting that you can choose from depending on your preferences and lifestyle. The three most common types of intermittent fasting are:

## Time-Restricted Eating:

This method involves eating only during a specific time window each day and fasting for the remaining hours. For example, you might choose to eat all of your meals between 12pm and 6pm and then fast for the remaining 18 hours of the day.

## Alternate-Day Fasting:

This method involves alternating between fasting days and eating days. On fasting days, you might consume only 500-600 calories, while on eating days, you can consume your regular calorie intake.

## The 16/8 Fasting Method:

also known as the time-restricted eating method, is a type of intermittent fasting that involves restricting your daily eating period to 8 hours and fasting for the remaining 16 hours. This method allows you to eat two or three meals within the 8-hour window, while avoiding food intake outside of the designated eating period. The 16/8 fasting method is one of the most popular types of intermittent fasting and can be easily integrated into your daily routine. It is recommended to start with shorter fasting periods and gradually increase the fasting window to 16 hours over time. This approach may help improve insulin sensitivity, aid in weight loss, and promote overall health and well-being.

**5:2 Diet:**

This method involves eating normally for five days of the week and restricting calories to 500-600 for two non-consecutive days of the week.

◆ ◆ ◆

When choosing the right type of intermittent fasting for you, it's important to consider your lifestyle and personal preferences. Time-restricted eating may be a good choice if you prefer a consistent routine and can stick to a specific eating window each day.

Alternate-day fasting may work well if you prefer a more flexible approach and can handle the hunger pangs on fasting days. The 5:2 diet may be a good choice if you want to ease into intermittent fasting and prefer to have a few days of regular eating each week.

It's also important to consider your health status and any medical conditions you may have. Some people may not be able to fast due to certain medical conditions, such as diabetes or pregnancy, and it's important to consult with a healthcare provider before starting any new diet or exercise program.

Ultimately, the best type of intermittent fasting for you is the one that you can sustain long-term and that fits into your lifestyle and goals. Experiment with different types of intermittent fasting and find the one that works best for you.

## *The potential risks and side effects of intermittent fasting*

While intermittent fasting can be a safe and effective way to improve overall health and manage weight, it is important to be aware of the potential risks and side effects.

One of the most common side effects of intermittent fasting is hunger pangs, especially during the initial stages of the fasting period. This can cause discomfort and make it challenging to stick to the fasting schedule. Another common side effect is fatigue or low energy, which can be attributed to the body adjusting to the new eating pattern.

Some people may also experience headaches, dizziness, or difficulty concentrating during the fasting period. These symptoms are usually temporary and will subside as the body adapts to the fasting schedule.

Intermittent fasting may not be suitable for everyone, especially those with certain health conditions such as diabetes, low blood pressure, or a history of disordered eating. It is important to consult a healthcare professional before starting any new dietary regimen, including intermittent fasting.

It is also important to ensure that you are consuming adequate nutrients and calories during your eating window to support overall health and prevent nutrient deficiencies.

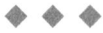

Overall, the potential risks and side effects of intermittent fasting can be managed by properly preparing for the fasting period, listening to your body, and seeking guidance from a healthcare professional if needed.

# STARTING YOUR 30-DAY INTERMITTENT FASTING JOURNEY

## *Tips, creating IF schedule and Setting Goals*

## *Tips for getting started with intermittent fasting*

If you are new to intermittent fasting, getting started can feel overwhelming. However, with the right mindset and approach, it can be a simple and sustainable lifestyle change. Here are some tips to help you get started with intermittent fasting:

**Start Slowly:**

Don't jump into a 24-hour fast right away. Start with a shorter fasting window, such as 12 hours, and gradually increase it over time.

**Choose A Fasting Plan That Works For You:**

Consider your lifestyle and choose a fasting plan that fits with your schedule and preferences. Some popular plans include the 16:8 method, the 5:2 method, and alternate-day fasting.

**Stay Hydrated:**

During your fasting window, it's important to stay hydrated. Drink plenty of water, herbal tea, or black coffee.

**Plan Your Meals:**

Plan your meals in advance, so you're not left hungry and tempted to break your fast with unhealthy food. Make sure to eat a balanced and nutritious meal during your eating window.

**Keep Busy:**

Staying busy can help you take your mind off of food and reduce feelings of hunger. Use your fasting window to tackle a project, exercise, or catch up on some reading.

## Be Kind To Yourself:

Remember, intermittent fasting is not a quick-fix solution. It's a lifestyle change that requires patience and persistence. Don't beat yourself up if you slip up or have a bad day. Just pick up where you left off and keep going.

## *Creating a fasting schedule that fits your lifestyle*

Creating a fasting schedule that fits your lifestyle is an important aspect of starting and maintaining an intermittent fasting practice. The schedule should be designed to suit your individual needs and preferences, while also ensuring that you can stick to the fasting protocol for the recommended duration.

There are several factors to consider when creating a fasting schedule, including the type of intermittent fasting protocol you have chosen, your work schedule, social obligations, and other lifestyle commitments.

For example, if you have chosen the 16/8 method, which involves fasting for 16 hours and eating within an 8-hour window, you may decide to skip breakfast and start your eating window at lunchtime. Alternatively, you could have an early dinner and fast until the next morning.

Another option is the 5:2 method, which involves eating normally for five days a week and restricting calorie intake to 500-600 calories on two non-consecutive days. You may choose to schedule your fasting days on weekdays when you are at work and can be distracted by tasks, while saving your non-fasting days for weekends or social events.

It is important to be realistic and flexible when creating a fasting schedule, as life can be unpredictable and certain situations may require adjustments. It may be helpful to start with a more lenient fasting schedule and gradually increase the duration and frequency of your fasts as your body adapts to the new routine.

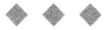

Overall, creating a fasting schedule that fits your lifestyle is key to the success of your intermittent fasting practice. It can help you to stay motivated, committed, and consistent with your fasting protocol, ultimately leading to improved health and wellness.

## *Setting realistic goals for your 30-day journey*

Setting realistic goals is an essential part of any health journey, including intermittent fasting. It's important to have clear and achievable goals in mind to help you stay motivated and on track during your 30-day intermittent fasting journey.

When setting goals for your fasting journey, it's important to consider your overall health and wellness goals. For example, do you want to lose weight, improve your blood sugar control, or reduce inflammation in your body?

Identifying your primary goals can help you choose the most appropriate type of intermittent fasting and create a fasting schedule that works for you.

It's also important to set realistic goals for your fasting schedule. For example, if you're new to fasting, it may not be realistic to start with a 24-hour fast. Instead, consider starting with a shorter fasting period, such as the 16/8 method, and gradually increasing the length of your fasts as you become more comfortable.

Another key consideration when setting goals is to be flexible and adaptable. Life can be unpredictable, and it's important to be able to adjust your fasting schedule to accommodate unexpected events or challenges.

Finally, it's important to celebrate your successes and acknowledge your progress along the way. Whether it's losing a few pounds, improving your energy levels, or feeling more focused and alert, taking time to recognize your accomplishments can help keep you motivated and committed to your health goals.

# NAVIGATING YOUR EATING WINDOW

*The What, The How and Meals*

## *What to eat during your eating window to optimize your health and weight loss goals*

During the eating window in intermittent fasting, it is important to focus on consuming nutrient-dense, whole foods that will support your health and weight loss goals. This means avoiding processed and high-calorie foods that are low in nutrients and may lead to overeating.

Here are some tips for what to eat during your eating window:

**Lean Proteins:**

Include sources of lean proteins such as chicken, turkey, fish, tofu, or legumes to help you feel full and support muscle growth.

**Whole Grains:**

Choose complex carbohydrates like brown rice, quinoa, or whole-wheat bread that will provide you with sustained energy and fiber.

**Fruits And Vegetables:**

Incorporate a variety of colorful fruits and vegetables to get essential vitamins, minerals, and antioxidants.

**Healthy Fats:**

Include sources of healthy fats such as avocado, nuts, seeds, and olive oil to help you feel satisfied and support heart health.

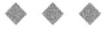

It's important to also pay attention to portion sizes and to not overeat during your eating window. Keep in mind that intermittent fasting is not a license to indulge in unhealthy foods, but rather a tool to promote a healthy and balanced diet.

*Recipes and meal ideas for a
healthy, balanced diet during
your eating window*

When it comes to meal planning during the eating window of intermittent fasting, it's important to focus on nutrient-dense, whole foods that will provide the energy and nourishment your body needs. Here are some recipe and meal ideas to consider:

**Breakfast:**

- Greek yogurt with berries and nuts
- Veggie omelet with spinach, tomatoes, and mushrooms
- Avocado toast with smoked salmon

**Lunch:**

- Grilled chicken salad with mixed greens, avocado, and tomatoes
- Turkey lettuce wraps with hummus and veggies
- Lentil soup with a side of roasted vegetables

**Dinner:**

- Baked salmon with roasted sweet potatoes and broccoli
- Grilled chicken with quinoa and roasted brussels sprouts
- Vegetarian chili with a side of cornbread

**Snacks:**

- Apple slices with almond butter
- Carrots and hummus
- Hard-boiled eggs

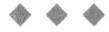

It's important to also pay attention to portion sizes and to listen to your body's hunger and fullness cues during the eating window. Drinking plenty of water throughout the day and staying hydrated can also help with cravings and hunger pangs.

## *How to handle cravings and hunger pangs during your fasting window*

Cravings and hunger pangs can be challenging to deal with during the fasting window of intermittent fasting. However, there are several strategies that can help individuals manage these sensations and stick to their fasting schedule.

Firstly, it is essential to ensure that you are consuming enough water throughout the day to stay hydrated. Drinking plenty of water can also help suppress hunger pangs and reduce cravings.

Another strategy to manage cravings and hunger pangs during the fasting window is to distract yourself with activities such as reading a book, taking a walk, or engaging in a hobby. These activities can take your mind off food and help you overcome the temporary sensations of hunger.

Additionally, it is important to consume a nutrient-dense meal before starting the fasting window. A meal that is high in fiber, protein, and healthy fats can help keep you feeling full for longer periods, reducing the likelihood of cravings or hunger pangs during the fasting period.

Lastly, it is important to remember that it is normal to experience some hunger during the fasting window, particularly when first starting with intermittent fasting. However, over time, the body can adjust to the new eating schedule, and hunger pangs may become less severe or frequent

# MAKING INTERMITTENT FASTING A SUSTAINABLE LIFESTYLE CHOICE

*How to continue, Strategies and the role of exercise in supporting the intermittent fasting*

# How to continue intermittent fasting beyond the 30-day period

Intermittent fasting can be a powerful tool for achieving better health and managing weight in the long-term. Once you have completed a 30-day intermittent fasting program, it's important to continue the practice in a sustainable way. Here are some tips for continuing intermittent fasting beyond the 30-day period:

## Gradually Increase Your Fasting Window:

If you started with a shorter fasting window, such as 12 hours, you can gradually increase it by 30 minutes or an hour each week until you reach your desired fasting window. This will give your body time to adjust to the longer fasting periods.

## Be Flexible With Your Fasting Schedule:

Life happens, and it's okay if you need to adjust your fasting schedule occasionally. For example, if you have a social event or a busy day at work, you can shift your fasting window to accommodate your schedule.

## Mix Up Your Fasting Methods:

Experiment with different types of intermittent fasting, such as the 5:2 method or alternate-day fasting, to keep your body from adapting to a single routine.

## Listen To Your Body:

If you feel fatigued, dizzy, or irritable during your fasting window, it may be a sign that you need to adjust your fasting schedule or the types of foods you eat during your eating window.

**Maintain A Healthy Diet:**

Even during your eating window, it's important to eat a balanced, nutritious diet that supports your health and weight loss goals. Focus on whole, unprocessed foods, plenty of vegetables, lean proteins, and healthy fats.

By following these tips, you can continue to reap the benefits of intermittent fasting in the long-term and maintain a healthy lifestyle.

## *Strategies for maintaining a healthy diet and lifestyle outside of your fasting window*

Maintaining a healthy diet and lifestyle outside of your fasting window is crucial for long-term success with intermittent fasting. Here are some strategies that can help:

**Choose Nutrient-Dense Foods:**

During your eating window, focus on consuming whole, nutrient-dense foods such as fruits, vegetables, lean proteins, and healthy fats. Avoid processed foods, sugary drinks, and snacks that are high in calories but low in nutrients.

**Plan Your Meals:**

Meal planning can help you stay on track and make healthy choices. Set aside some time each week to plan your meals and snacks, and make a grocery list to ensure you have everything you need.

**Mindful Eating:**

Mindful eating means paying attention to your hunger and fullness cues, and enjoying your food without distractions. This can help you avoid overeating and make more conscious food choices.

**Stay Hydrated:**

Drinking plenty of water throughout the day can help you stay hydrated and may help reduce feelings of hunger during your fasting period.

**Exercise Regularly:**

Regular exercise can help support weight loss and overall health. Incorporate a mix of aerobic exercise and strength training into your routine.

**Get Enough Sleep:**

Adequate sleep is essential for maintaining a healthy weight and reducing the risk of chronic diseases. Aim for 7-9 hours of sleep each night to support your health goals.

**Practice Self-Care:**

Taking care of your mental and emotional health is just as important as physical health. Find activities that help you relax and reduce stress, such as meditation, yoga, or reading a book.

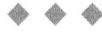

Remember, intermittent fasting is not a magic bullet for weight loss and overall health. It is one tool in your toolbox to support your goals. Maintaining a healthy diet and lifestyle outside of your fasting window is essential for long-term success.

## *The role of exercise in supporting intermittent fasting and overall health*

Exercise plays a crucial role in supporting intermittent fasting and overall health. Regular physical activity has numerous health benefits, such as improving heart health, increasing muscle mass, reducing stress, and improving sleep quality. When combined with intermittent fasting, exercise can also help to optimize weight loss, improve metabolic health, and enhance overall well-being.

It is important to choose an exercise routine that fits with your fasting schedule and lifestyle. For example, if you are following the 16/8 fasting method and skip breakfast, you may want to schedule your workout during your fasting window to maximize fat burning potential. Alternatively, if you prefer to exercise in the morning, you may want to adjust your fasting schedule accordingly.

A combination of both cardio and strength training is recommended for optimal health and weight loss benefits. Cardiovascular exercise such as running, cycling, or swimming can help to burn calories and improve cardiovascular health. Strength training, such as weight lifting, resistance band exercises, or bodyweight exercises, can help to build muscle mass and increase metabolism.

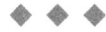

It is important to listen to your body and not push yourself too hard, especially during the early stages of intermittent fasting. If you are feeling weak or dizzy during exercise, it may be a sign that your body needs more fuel. Be sure to stay hydrated and fuel your body with nutritious foods during your eating window to support your exercise routine and overall health.

# TROUBLESHOOTING COMMON CHALLENGES AND ROADBLOCKS

*Overcoming common challenges,*
*Strategies and Tips*

## *How to overcome common challenges such as social events, travel, and work schedules*

Intermittent fasting can present some challenges when it comes to social events, travel, and work schedules. However, there are some strategies that can help individuals stay on track with their fasting goals even in these situations.

**Social Events:**

When attending social events such as dinners or parties, it is important to plan ahead. Consider eating a small meal or snack before the event to help curb hunger and avoid overeating later. Choose foods that are higher in protein and fiber, such as vegetables or lean protein sources, to help keep you feeling full longer. Alternatively, consider adjusting your fasting schedule for the day to allow for a later eating window that aligns with the event.

**Travel:**

Travel can disrupt regular eating and fasting schedules, but it is still possible to maintain a fasting routine while on the road. Pack healthy snacks such as nuts, fruits, or protein bars to help curb hunger during long flights or car rides. Choose restaurants that offer healthy options, such as salads or grilled lean meats, and adjust your fasting schedule as needed to fit your travel itinerary.

**Work Schedules:**

Some work schedules may make it challenging to stick to a

consistent fasting routine. If you work long hours or have irregular shift work, consider adjusting your fasting schedule to accommodate your work schedule. Plan your meals and snacks in advance and bring them with you to work to avoid impulsive food choices or temptations.

Ultimately, the key to overcoming common challenges during intermittent fasting is to plan ahead and be flexible. Don't be too hard on yourself if you miss a fasting period or have to adjust your schedule to accommodate unexpected events. Remember that intermittent fasting is a lifestyle choice and it is important to find a routine that works best for your individual needs and goals.

## *Strategies for dealing with hunger, low energy, and other side effects of intermittent fasting*

Intermittent fasting can cause hunger, low energy, and other side effects, especially when first starting out. Here are some strategies to help deal with these issues:

**Stay Hydrated:**

Drink plenty of water, unsweetened tea, or other calorie-free beverages to help curb hunger and maintain energy levels.

**Eat Nutrient-Dense Foods:**

Choose whole, nutrient-dense foods that provide sustained energy, such as lean protein, complex carbohydrates, and healthy fats. Avoid processed and high-sugar foods that can cause energy crashes.

**Incorporate Healthy Snacks:**

If you find yourself feeling too hungry during your fasting window, incorporate healthy snacks like fresh fruits, nuts, or vegetables to help keep you feeling full and energized.

**Gradually Increase Fasting Time:**

If you are experiencing hunger or low energy during fasting, try gradually increasing your fasting time by 15 or 30 minutes each day until you reach your desired fasting schedule.

**Experiment With Meal Timing And Composition:**

Try different meal timing and composition strategies, such as eating larger meals during your eating window or incorporating more healthy fats to help you feel full and satisfied.

**Get Enough Sleep:**

Getting adequate sleep is crucial for maintaining energy levels and managing hunger. Aim for 7-9 hours of quality sleep per night.

**Manage Stress:**

Stress can cause hunger and affect energy levels. Incorporate stress-management techniques like meditation, yoga, or deep breathing exercises to help manage stress levels.

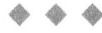

It's important to note that some people may experience more severe side effects of intermittent fasting, such as dizziness, headaches, or nausea. If you experience any of these symptoms, it may be best to consult with a healthcare professional before continuing with intermittent fasting.

## *What to do if you are not seeing the desired results from your fasting journey*

If you are not seeing the desired results from your fasting journey, it's important to first reassess your fasting schedule and diet to make sure you are following them correctly. Sometimes, small adjustments can make a big difference. Here are some other strategies to consider:

### Track Your Food Intake:

Keep a food diary or use a tracking app to monitor your daily food intake. This can help you identify areas where you may be consuming too many calories or not getting enough of certain nutrients.

### Adjust Your Fasting Schedule:

If you're not seeing results, you may want to try adjusting your fasting schedule. For example, you could try extending your fasting window, shortening your eating window, or switching to a different type of intermittent fasting.

### Focus On Nutrient-Dense Foods:

Make sure you are eating a variety of nutrient-dense foods, such as lean proteins, vegetables, fruits, and healthy fats. These foods will help you feel fuller longer and provide your body with the nutrients it needs to function optimally.

**Increase Your Physical Activity:**

Exercise is an important part of any weight loss or health program. Try increasing your activity level by incorporating more movement into your daily routine, such as taking the stairs instead of the elevator or going for a walk after dinner.

**Consider Seeking Professional Guidance:**

If you're still not seeing results or are experiencing other health issues, consider seeking the guidance of a registered dietitian or healthcare professional who can help you develop a personalized plan that works for you.

# CONCLUSION

# EPILOGUE

Congratulations! You have completed the 30-day intermittent fasting journey and have taken a significant step towards achieving your health and wellness goals. This book was designed to guide you through the science behind intermittent fasting, different types of fasting schedules, and strategies to help you navigate your fasting and eating windows.

As you continue on your health and wellness journey, it's important to remember that intermittent fasting is just one part of a healthy lifestyle. Consistency and moderation are key, so don't be too hard on yourself if you slip up occasionally.

Remember to continue making healthy food choices during your eating window, stay hydrated, and incorporate physical activity into your daily routine. You can also experiment with different fasting schedules to find the one that works best for you and your lifestyle.

Most importantly, celebrate your achievements and progress, no matter how small they may seem. You have taken a significant step towards improving your health and well-being, and that's something to be proud of.

❖ ❖ ❖

Thank you for choosing this book as your guide on your intermittent fasting journey. I wish you continued success on your health and wellness journey!

# ACKNOWLEDGEMENT

I would like to express my deep appreciation to all of the people who helped me bring this book to fruition. First and foremost, I want to thank my family for their unwavering support and encouragement throughout this journey. I also want to thank my editor, who provided valuable feedback and guidance throughout the writing process.

A special thanks goes out to the experts and professionals who contributed their knowledge and experience to this book. Your insights and expertise were invaluable in creating a comprehensive guide to intermittent fasting.

I would also like to thank my readers, whose interest and enthusiasm for the subject matter continue to inspire me. Your feedback and comments have been invaluable in shaping the final product.

Finally, I want to acknowledge the thousands of individuals who have embraced the practice of intermittent fasting and shared their stories of success and transformation. Your courage and dedication serve as a constant source of inspiration and motivation.

www.ingramcontent.com/pod-product-compliance
Lightning Source LLC
Chambersburg PA
CBHW071113220526
45467CB00004B/1856